TANTRIC SEX POSITIONS

INCREASE INTIMACY AND YOUR OVERALL SEXUAL LIFE

Victor E.Sellner

© Copyright 2021 - All rights reserved.

The content contained within this book may not be reproduced, duplicated or transmitted without direct written permission from the author or the publisher.

Under no circumstances will any blame or legal responsibility be held against the publisher, or author, for any damages, reparation, or monetary loss due to the information contained within this book. Either directly or indirectly.

Legal Notice:

This book is copyright protected. This book is only for personal use. You cannot amend, distribute, sell, use, quote or paraphrase any part, or the content within this book, without the consent of the author or publisher.

Disclaimer Notice:

Please note the information contained within this document is for educational and entertainment purposes only. All effort has been executed to present accurate, up to date, and reliable, complete information. No warranties of any kind are declared or implied. Readers acknowledge that the author is not engaging in the rendering of legal, financial, medical or professional advice. The content within this book has been derived from various sources. Please consult a licensed professional before attempting any techniques outlined in this book.

By reading this document, the reader agrees that under no circumstances is the author responsible for any losses, direct or indirect, which are incurred as a result of the use of information contained within this document, including, but not limited to, errors, omissions, or inaccuracies.

Table Of Contents

INTRODUCTION	6
CHAPTER 1: WHAT IS TANTRA?	10
BUDDHISM AND TANTRIC SEX	11
WHAT ABOUT NEOTANTRA	12
CHAPTER 2: HISTORY AND ORIGIN OF TANTRA	16
THE ORIGIN OF TANTRA	17
THE TANTRA TEXTS	19
HOW DID TANTRA ARRIVE IN THE WEST	22
TANTRA AND THE WAY OF LIBERATION	22
CHAPTER 3: BENEFITS OF TANTRIC SEX	24
CHAPTER 4: THE TANTRA OF LOVE	28
OPENING OF THE HOLY CHAKRA	30
TANTRIC SEXUAL EXPERIENCE IS DIVIDED INTO THREE STAGES	31
MYTHS AND THE TRUTHS ABOUT TANTRIC SEX AND TANTRA	37
CHAPTER 5: YANTRA	40
OPERATION OF YANTRAS	41
TYPES OF YANTRAS USED IN TANTRIC PRACTICES	42
HOW TO USE YANTRAS IN TANTRIC PRACTICES	44
CHAPTER 6: MANTRA	46
YOGA AND MANTRA	47
SANSKRIT AND MANTRA	47
REFLECTION AND MANTRA	48
YOGA AND OM SHANTI	50
CHAPTER 7: YIN & YANG	56
SHIVA AND SHAKTI	57
UNDERSTANDING THE OPPOSITES	58
MY PARTNER IS MY BELOVED	59
THE DESIRE SPECTRUM	59
YOU FEEL EMPOWERED TO SAY WHAT YOU WANT!	60
CHAPTER 8: TANTRIC COMMUNICATION	62
WHY ARE SUCH A LOT OF HUMANS TURNING TO TANTRA TO CLEAR UP THEIR DATING CHALLENGES?	68
DIVINE LOVE MEDITATION	69

CHAPTER 9: TANTRIC MASSAGE AND TANTRIC YOGA 72
Benefits of Tantric Massage 73

CHAPTER 10: TANTRIC SEX POSITIONS 84
The Sidewinder 84
The Yab Yum 85
The Latch 86
The Butterfly 87
The Double Decker 88
The Last Place Anyone Would Want to Be 89
Skiff 90
The Mermaid 91
Tsunami 92
Lap Dance 93
Pretzel 94
The Spread 95
The Entwine 96
The G-force 97
The Waterfall 98
The Snake 99

CHAPTER 11: MULTIPLE ORGASM 100
Benefits of Orgasms 101
Types of Orgasm 102
The Female Orgasm 103
The Male Orgasm 105
Multiple Orgasms 106

CHAPTER 12: TIPS TO IMPROVE TANTRIC SEX 110

CONCLUSION 118

INTRODUCTION

In the Tantric tradition, specific physical positions, which enhance the mind-body connection and promote more profound states of consciousness, are employed for sexual intercourse. The parts are believed to influence the development and progress of diseases. Most of these Tantric sex positions are based on the Muladhara or Base Chakra, located at the lowest point in the spine, representing the ground of their being or the concrete base the couple has in the physical world.

Like the other Tantric positions, these positions are part of the Tantric tradition, which can be traced back to the Hindu traditions' kama sutra and the Taoist teachings of China that both seek to harness sexual energy attain a state of physical, mental, and spiritual well-being.

These positions are designed to create a meditative and spiritual experience by prolonging the sexual act and merging with the sexual energy– for both the man and the woman. Although it is not physically possible for the man to satisfactorily indulge in both of these Tantric sex positions whilst being penetrated, he can however perform the same motions in a similar way to the woman, which benefits him greatly.

Tantric sex for the Tantric Buddhists focuses their attention on the Muladhara or Base Chakra. Tantra (Sanskrit, meaning "loom") is the term used to describe a yoga method that originated in ancient India and focuses on using sexual energy or desire to attain liberation and achieve spiritual interconnectedness. The word "tantra" itself means "to expand, to weave, extend, and be ingenious, skillful." Tantric Buddhism was brought to Tibet by the great Indian sage Padmasambhava, also known as Guru Rinpoche, in the 8th century. It is considered the most advanced form of Buddhism and is regarded as the core of Vajrayana Buddhism. Tantric Buddhists focus on touching and being touched in areas such as the genitals, which allows for more profound levels of intimacy and spiritual connection. This sexual energy is then purified to the central channel through meditation, enabling a state of ecstatic unity with nature.

The Hindu yogis most likely brought the physical positions and meditation techniques. Some contemporary has found that these practices influenced the early religious movements in Tibet like the great Mahayana Buddhist teachers. They were responsible for the introduction of Chorten, or mountain temples. From the local Hindu yogis in Western India, adept at Tantric meditation and other techniques, they introduced these practices into Tibet and China, which then spread abroad from the Himalayan region.

The Tibetan monks are commonly celibate, but the Tibetan lamas, the highest religious authority, are not required to be so. But at the same time, they maintain a vow of chastity as a sign of their spiritual commitment to superior beings. Currently, there are over 100,000 Tibetan monks who have taken full ordination within the Buddhist religion.

Bringing this into contemporary times, the Chinese Taoist teachings, which are hundreds of years old, teach that the man and woman are uniting in lovemaking embrace Yin and Yang's exchange or male and female energies. The joining of these opposite energies serves several purposes. First of all, it helps achieve a healthy body if the points are balanced, and secondly, it supports the attainment of spiritual freedom or enlightenment by the intensification of awareness. The sexual energy is conducted through the meridians, which are channels in the body that join the organs and the body's surface. The point is made to travel through the body, which allows for deep relaxation of the physical, mental, emotional, and spiritual organs. Achieving this heightened sense of awareness is the goal of this growth process into becoming a powerful being who can achieve real spiritual connection and achieve enlightenment.

CHAPTER 1:

WHAT IS TANTRA?

Tantra is a part of tantric sex, but tantric sex comes from both tantra and neotantra. Tantra is something that's found in advanced Hindu teachings, along with Buddhist and other Asian teachings. Tantra is something that's been around for many years, and it's an ancient ritualistic practice that involves practitioners, and close direction of the person who is guiding them, called a guru. Not as many people practice this form for a good reason. The typical tantric sex that we know about that doesn't require a guru and isn't as ritualistic is neotantra. This was recently imported to the western countries, and it's only partially taken from the religious roots, so it's not as religious in practice as typical tantra. It's often called modern tantra or called "California tantra," but this is a derogatory term. This is often viewed as sexual practices together as a whole, not just sexual intercourse. This is typically used for more intimacy, and to help provide an orgasm that's more delayed and or powerful not just for themselves but also their partner. However, there is also tantric sex within Hinduism, and there are a few interesting aspects of it.

Buddhism and Tantric Sex

Tantric sex was used in Vajrayana Buddhism, and this one is a very advanced form of Buddhism, but it still has 10 million adherents to it, and two schools mostly focused on this. You can find this in Mongolia, China, Nepal, Russia, India, Tibet, and Japan for the most part.

One of the main goals of Buddhism, however, is to overcome your desire. This was the idea that the best way to achieve this was to experience passion, and from there, try to train it so you can control this.

His idea was that the people who were on his pathway would do this to attain enlightenment. They might be restricted for a while and practice tantric sex to experience the culture, rather than mere pleasure.

It did adopt the Hindu idea that the energy centers within the body, which are the chakras that are there, could be activated and released. The goal is to get the chakra at the crown of the head, which is where spiritual evolution is, and from there, transform your consciousness, and ultimately reach for nirvana.

The Buddhist traditions might use sexual yoga to magnify and move the energy that's innate within them. This does have orgasms, of course, but it doesn't have just pleasure-seeking ideas behind this. Often, the sexual energy is then deflected to the mystical channel that focuses on enlightenment rather than mere pleasure.

Of course, this practice isn't without danger s. Sometimes, you might use these techniques to achieve orgasm, or by getting the methods and sharing them with people who shouldn't know, that could result in mental illness, or you may have rebirth cycles in hell due to this.

Again, this tantric practice is ritualistic in aspects of putting your life in order and putting you in synch with nature as well. The idea behind this is to ritualize yourself from the moment you get up, during the day, as you go to bed, and when you're sleeping until you wake up the next day. You don't even have to use sexual yoga to practice tantra, but instead, you try to practice restraint and understanding.

What about NeoTantra

Neotantra is that hybrid of both of these, where it combines a lot of the tantra styles of both.

It's imported for the most part, and it uses the traditional yoga positions, along with meditation and breath control. Still, it's taught outside of the Hindu religion and culture, and you don't have to be religious to do it.

Some people also incorporate massages into this, including tantric massages, bioenergetics, counseling, and sexual healing. You sometimes need to learn a course of study for a couple of these areas, but the average person can utilize tantric sex and benefit from it.

The goal that is sought by the person differs each time. Rather than just a state of tantric bliss like thin the other types of tantras, it pushes for more intimacy with one another, along with the delayed and amazingly intensified orgasm. The neotantra practice focuses much more on sex and having better orgasms, whereas the traditional tantra does not.

Tantra is excellent, but it's hard, and many times they focus much more on self-restraint. Neo-tantra is more about having fun, but they may not focus on the other tantric practices you might get from traditional tantra.

Neotantra has the connections to the new-age spiritual practices, but not always, but sometimes it does contain other forms of sacred sexuality too, and sometimes is used for advertising sexual education course s to others.

Some commercial sex workers will use this as a gimmick, too, to increases their sales. It does modify both the Hindu and the Buddhist tantra idea by getting rid of where the guru is involved and getting rid of the extensive and intensive meditation it otherwise calls for.

So why are people attracted to it? Well, I promise fulfillment and excitement while you stimulate your natural sexual impulses, along with the neurotic needs that you have emotionally, with a hint of spirituality. The cool thing about modern tantra is that you can learn all about all of the different ceremonies and philosophies, and they can be used to promote the tantra mentality.

The Kamasutra and the Anga Ranga are also a part of this in a sense, since it applies to these sutras, or positions, to accommodate for love along with sex that doesn't happen in traditional tantras.

The traditional tantra is excellent to understand and has some sexual elements at the core, but you need to realize that it's more than just that. It's just replicating the feelings of sex, love, and wellness in both a physical and spiritual form, bringing about a better understanding of the other person.

These different types of tantras are entirely valid, and neotantra is a good practice, but you should learn the difference between all of these. The tantra roots are ancient, and this older form is still handy. It's just adopted a modern concept for you to use.

CHAPTER 2:

HISTORY AND ORIGIN OF TANTRA

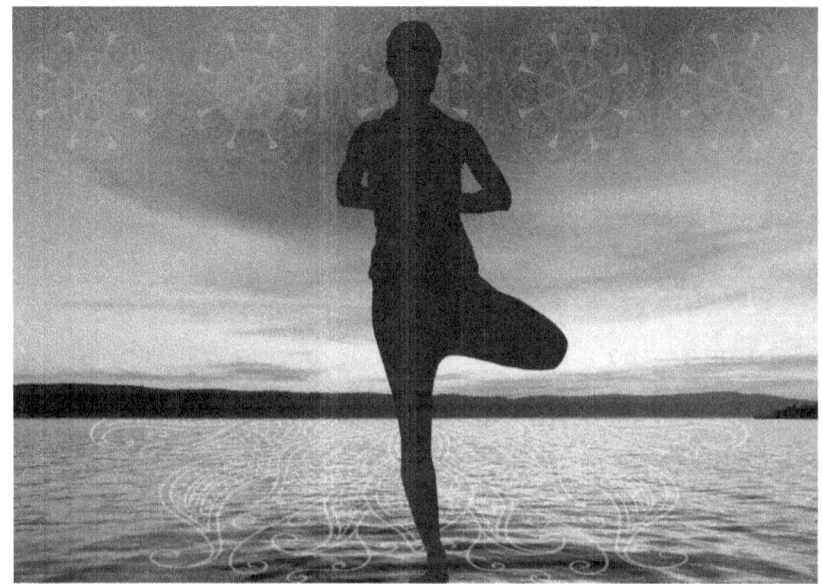

The original tantra, also called "red" or "left hand," is linked to ancient matriarchal societies and has female energy as its center. While the Tantra called "White" or "right-handed," created later due to Muslim infiltrations, derives from Indian patriarchal societies.

The difference between Red Tantra and White Tantra is radical. The second, White Tantra, is based on static and solitary meditations, while Red Tantra is a practice in which meditation is not just immobility and seriousness. In Red Tantra, meditation and sacredness are experienced in every moment of existence, through deep listening and attention to what is happening in us and outside of us. Reflection occurs while dancing, working, embracing, eating, drinking, playing, and talking. There is a lot of confusion about what Tantra is and, above all, a lot of targeted misinformation due to the persecutions to which the Original Tantra was subjected. Tantra carries the burden of false commonplaces, such as that of free sex. Unlike other disciplines that have been less polluted, Tantra is for many a kind of Yoga practice; for others, an orgiastic approach and for still others a religion.

The Origin of Tantra

According to the almost unanimous opinion of scholars, the archaic nature of Red Tantra dates back to pre-Vedic cultures, to the very beginnings of Indian history, identifiable with the Harappei, Sindhu, and other Dravidian populations which developed their civilization in the Indus valley. According to some, in the third millennium BC, these populations were widespread in a vast territory from Spain to the Ganges valley. Their precursors had settled in the Indus valley in Mehrgar, starting from 7000 BC, and their traces can be found up to 5500 BC.

Dravidian populations, therefore, appeared there around 6000-5000 BC, had their apogee between 2300 and 1300 BC., and disappeared, rather quickly, in 100 years between 1900 and 1800 BC. The disappearance's reasons were attributed in the past to invasions of the Arii population from the north. Today there is a tendency to attribute it instead to a tectonic movement that caused the Aravali hills in northern Rajastan to rise, depriving the river that supported the Dravida civilization (the Ghaggar-Hakra) of most of its tributaries.

The Harappei population showed a significant interest in the arts and well-being. Theirs was a matriarchal society, the most critical central monument of their city. It was a large swimming pool; the water element was fundamental in their organization, and there has already been a bathroom in every home. The woman was at the center of culture, focused on the mother goddess. The female figure dominated the sanctuaries and, with open arms and legs, offered herself to adoration. The Harappei used to keep a large bed in the center of the essential room in the house and practiced Tantra. Their religion was closely connected with the body, well-being, and sexuality.

It can be said that Red Tantra is the expression of all those practices, which also include sexuality. Red Tantra contains methods carried out in groups, including contact and "vehiculation" through the senses.

In the centuries following the birth of Tantra, in India, due to the Islamic invasions, the original Red Tantra was officially suppressed and forced to transform itself into an occult school. Today we know it as Tantra Yoga, and it has completely lost its peculiarity of a concrete approach to sexuality, typical of the original Tantra.

In practice, the White Tantra is a Red Tantra but censored by all those practices that moralists could understand as unbecoming. Today the White Tantra, which is, therefore, a mystification of the original Tantra, is used in the West for commercial purposes. Almost all Tantra schools practice White Tantra and therefore do not teach Tantra.

Authentic Tantra is the way of reconnection with one's self. It is the way; that of discovering our genotypic sexual energies that are manifested through the knowledge and practice of the Original Tantra.

The Tantra Texts

The Tantras are a series of texts of Central Asian origin (India, Kashmir, Bengal, Orissa, Assam, Kerala, Indus Valley, etc.) like the collections of the Puranas or the Vedas, but which manifest themselves in the manner of esoteric texts divine revealed and are often written as if they were the gods Shiva and Shakty (and their emanations) in-person speaking and are part of the Hindu Texts Agama.

The origin of the Tantras is pre-Vedic, which is much older than the texts on which Hinduism and the Vedas are based, and originates from the ancient matriarchal peoples and, in general, all the collections of Hindu texts are deeply influenced by the Tantra. No Hindu and Brahmin ritual does not have its roots in Tantra.

The Tantras were transcribed long after their birth, as previously the tradition was handed down only orally from master to teacher, from teacher to teacher. In fact, in Tantra, unlike Hinduism, the teachers could be men or women. Starting from about the VI AD instead, the written transcriptions of many Tantras begin to appear.

Tantric texts have more than one reading and can be experienced at different levels of intuition. According to the Tantric tradition, a text can confuse or illuminate. Tantric texts often speak by aphorisms (sutra and karika) and often then generate immense commentaries that explain aphorisms that can sometimes be difficult to understand.

The term Tantra, linked to the ancient texts, was then translated also to indicate the Spiritual Experiential Way that follows these ancient teachings.

More than 500 existing Tantras are known which belong to different initiatory ways or lineages. Many of them have never even been translated from Sanskrit. Other tantric texts have been lost, and it is not known what they handed down. It is said that the books reached a considerable number of 14000 volumes. So, the panorama of tantric initiatory texts is very vast, and not all Tantras treat themes equally according to the lineage to which they belong. So, this also generates some confusion regarding the teachings. Some Tantric Texts can be of a few pages, others of thousands of pages. It should therefore be understood that different teachings are grouped under the word Tantra, although on many points, many Tantra essentially agrees. It cannot be said that the various tantric texts contradict each other, but that they simply give certain importance more to one aspect than to another. Some Tantras favor the transmission of the concept of presence, others of the concept of the body, others concerning sexuality. A generally shared aspect is the "freed in life," that is, the unnecessary need for countless reincarnations to dissolve Karma. In fact, in tantra, it is indicated that by following certain rituals or teachings, it is possible to dissolve the karmic knots quickly, soon arriving at a knowledge of oneself also through the experimentation of eros and sexuality in the encounter between Shiva and Shakti and in any case following a way away from the renunciation of the body. The revelations of the Tantras are considered superior to the Vedas because they are much more effective in the liberation of men and lead them faster to a higher stage and are more suitable for the current cosmic era, the Kaliyuga. Tantra considers the Vedic texts to be valid, but on a lower level as basic general rules, but which are then integrated by higher and esoteric specific tantric teachings. Tantric texts do not address the renunciation ascetic of the world, but on the contrary, they address those who live in the world, together with others, without going away or dedicating themselves to asceticism.

How did Tantra Arrive in the West

In conjunction with the sexual liberation of the 60s and 70s and the emancipation of women, some scholars and philosophers began to talk about Tantra and trying to make it a practicable approach even in the West, made the rituals more agile and less blocking in the calculation of breath and holding of positions. Currently, emancipation allows women to get closer to the sexual world, although, in western society, it is still believed that sex is more masculine than feminine, and cultural heritage does not allow women to focus on that.

In the West today, Tantra aims to draw two maps, one that indicates how to make the sexual experience spiritual and how to unite the earth with the sky, in a terrain where separation and judgment vanish. A world, the western one, where there are no schools and traditions, and everything is to be invented and experimented with. In the West, the sexual sphere has been a world crushed for two millennia by taboos and religions, which often finds its only expression in private clubs or porn sites.

Tantra and the Way of Liberation

With all its erotic experiences, Tantra is nothing more than a tool that opens up internal physical, emotional, and energetic spaces and opens up to awareness. Tantra is, therefore, only Red Tantra. It is the way of liberation that opens up to the true expression of oneself, and that allows one to exit, both in the imaginary and in the real, from the dimension of the matrix in which sexual energy is mechanically channeled for improper purposes.

Sex and sexual energy are very different things. The idea of sex is what in the imagination has settled during education, stories, and commercial pornography, a program, therefore, but so rooted that individuals believe that it is precisely that pre-programmed way that sexual energy must be expressed. A program that is then gradually enhanced with the repetitive experiences that add up as memories.

The vital energy or commonly known as sexual energy (Kundalini), is instead what is the essence of the man at its origin; it is what we carry in our genes, but which, due to the education received in the matrix, is then unnaturally expressed in the facts.

Over time, with the help of religious morality, the matrix selected a sexual modality aimed entirely at procreation, therefore mechanical and centered on penetration and orgasm intended as a goal to be achieved; as if all the wonder of the contact between the bodies should be enclosed in the act of a few minutes, between the two genital organs. Many people believe they are sexually free because they do a lot of that mechanical sex, while in reality, they are just more slaves; slaves to a trap where true sexual energy is humiliated and crushed.

CHAPTER 3:

BENEFITS OF TANTRIC SEX

You have encountered several benefits of practicing tantric sex. Yet, you will notice a vast difference in these new ones despite their interconnection. Those are not the only benefits you gain as you try tantric sex. There are more in wait for you.

1. **Expansion of Love Possibility:** With tantric sex, you are sure to expand the possibility of gaining love or deepening the love you and your partner have. It also would increase the spiritual connections that would allow you to adore your partner and still find yourself worthy of love.

2. **Health Rejuvenation:** The psychological and physiological effect that comes with tantric sex is sure to keep you in good health. They not only maintain good health but also help you in regaining poor ones.

    Take the breathing techniques you will learn later as an example. It will help you improve the way you breathe, thus giving your body more room to take in more air. This process will nourish your body tissues and muscles.

Research shows that when we relax, meditate, or go on spiritual exercise, we are sure to improve our emotional and physical health. Spiritual people are sure to have lower blood pressure and less likely to be anxious or depressed. Not only those, but they will also have stable hormone levels. Invariably, their immune system will function better.

3. **Youthfulness:** Tantra allows you to tap into the fountain of youth. Since your body will not age quickly due to having healthy blood pressure, you are assured of the different things at your disposal to ensure you are looking young.

4. **Women Empowerment:** You were not waiting for that. But women are sure to suffer low-esteem about their bodies. Sometimes, they are careful about saying their sexual need because of this low self-esteem. But when you try tantric sex with your partner, the esteems of both individuals are skyrocketed because the body is treated with respect and honor. They feel desired and deserving.

5. **Empowers Men:** The two major problems faced with sex are the penis length and their longevity in bed. This has always ruined the experience because they are always looking inward instead of their partners' needs. They are also poor at pleasing women in bed because

they focus on staying long instead of enjoying sex. When they don't focus on the women, they tend to displease the women more. Tantric sex is opening both parties to great satisfaction; thus, giving the man high esteem for his body.

6. **Great Sexual Satisfaction:** No doubt, sex has always left several people feeling they are not done. They want more and were left hanging in the balance because their sex was more genital-centric. The sexual connection didn't touch the heart or the soul. Tantric sex will help you make the heart feel the love and make the body feel more nurtured because of the soul connection you feel with your partner. As soon as the heart is fed with substantial sexual, the body and mind would enjoy the meal.

7. **Anxieties and Depression Alleviation:** One thing is sure, tantric sex will help in alleviating your anxiety and depression level. From statistics, several millions of people are battling anxiety and depression, which indicate that they suffer from such things as fatigue, restlessness, and sleeping/eating disturbance. You are sure to enjoy enormous positive energy from tantric sex that will improve the peacefulness of your body.

8. **Elevates Sex:** When sex is upped to a state of sacredness, then you are sure to enjoy a more luxurious dimension to it. This elevation would make regular sex seems wrong.

9. **Prolong Pleasure:** Tantric sex is simply upgraded lovemaking, which means there would be an extreme level of afterglow. This glow is sure to be on the increase because of the ejaculatory control and the way you directed your sexual energy in the spiritual manifestations.

10. **Healing:** As shown before, there are several ways tantric sex can heal you. Tantric sex will leave you with the feeling of being honored and respected in sex and life.

11. **Deepen Your Connection to Others:** Your self-esteem has been improved that you have little to worry about as regards yourself. This will make you stop worrying about yourself and start actually caring for people. Your connection to them will genuinely deepen.

12. **Be Relevant to the World:** Since you are no longer buried in yourself, your eyes are opened to the mysteries in the earth. Your energy will alter the energy of the planet in a positive way. People are now feeling positive and are also generating good feelings about themselves.

CHAPTER 4:

The Tantra of Love

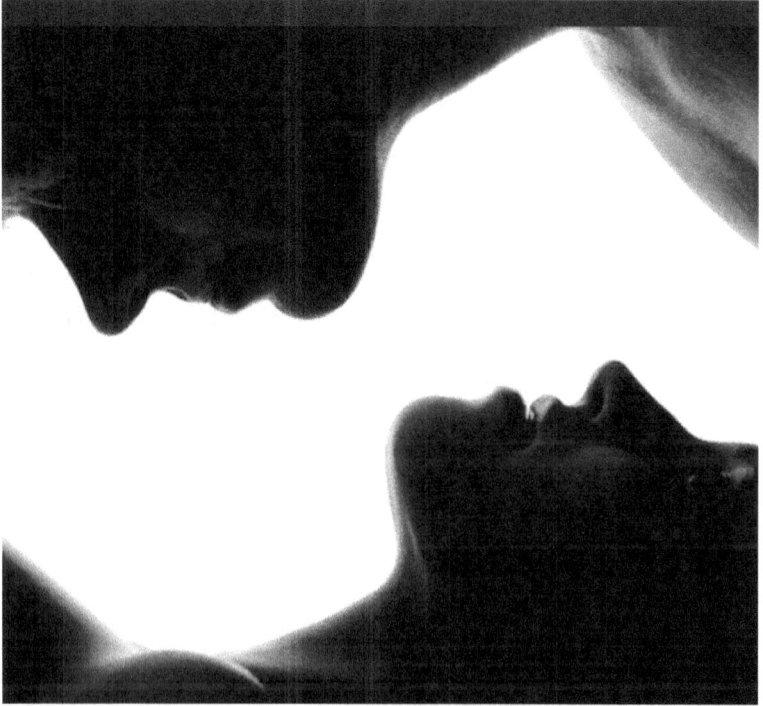

Tantra is the oldest sacred art of sexuality known to humanity and is still practiced to this day. However, the origin of the Tantra is not clear. There are different versions, including one that says Tantra is a disciplined Hindu system. Other historians say that Tantra comes from Buddhist monks. Still, others claim that Tantra was developed from rural communities in East India. There are other so-called experts who believe that yoga and tantra are one and the same. However, the key goal of yoga is to cultivate self-awareness and higher consciousness, while Tantra is about weaving and releasing the body. Considering the fact that most of the physically difficult positions of tantric sex are known from yoga positions, these experts have concluded that even if tantra is not yoga, it is modeled on yoga. The modern world knows about Tantra is that its most common form has retained some of the popular ancient writings, such as Kama Sutra (allegedly in Christ's day) and Anang Rank (a collection of erotic writings, first published in 1100 AD). A nobleman would be the author of the Kama Sutra. He saw life as involving dharma or a spiritual substance, artha or financial substance, and Kama, or sensual substance.

The Kama is known as "enjoying the right objects by the five senses, aided by the mind and soul." Tantra may seem like the art of sexual pleasure, and Kama Sutra is a set of sexual positions. Kama's main goal is to cultivate love and develop worship and reverence for his partner's body.

Looking at the tantric experience, it is easy to assume that you will have "great sex." However, if it is seen and experienced outside of the physical aspect (with clairvoyance), then it is, in fact, amazing dance and show of colors and energy, like the "epic experience of fireworks."

Opening of the Holy Chakra

To prepare for tantric sex, you must first learn to open the sacred chakra. To do this, follow the instructions below:

- Spend time near open waters and in the moonlight. It will help you feel and appreciate the healthy flow mechanisms in your own body.

- Try to surround yourself with beauty. For example, flowers, color, art, and music - or anything else that makes you happy and even more appreciative of your role in this world.

- Try using fragrances with sandalwood, musk, or ylang-ylang. They open the Holy Chakra more than any other perfume.

You can also repeat the following statements:

- I allow myself to enjoy my sexuality.

- I know that pleasure is an important and sacred part of my life.

- The opportunity to enjoy sex and sensuality brings me joy and nourishes my spirit.

- Let me fill my emotions well.

- My life is pleasant and graceful.

Tantric Sexual Experience is Divided into Three Stages

1. Physical

The main emphasis is on the physical pleasure that you feel at this particular time.

Here are some of the ways that can help you experience physical tantric sex:

- **Stop Talking**

    Just get lost right now. Privacy is not just dirty conversations; Sometimes it's also about silence - how will you allow yourself to focus only on the moment and not think or talk about anything for a few minutes (preferably even longer).

- **Try to Slow Down**

    Undress. Focus on every part of the body, instead of being brutal right away. To enjoy the beauty of intimacy, you need to learn every part of your partner's body. You must appreciate the beauty of undressing and the joy of foreplay. Take your time - there's nothing wrong with that.

- **Enjoy Sex without Orgasms**

    Sometimes you become intimate just because you can't wait for orgasm. Learn to enjoy foreplay and understand that even without orgasm, sex can be an incredibly beautiful experience for you and your partner.

- **Give Him Life**

    This means that you also need to focus on breathing you and your partner. Hearing your partner's breathing sound can be sexy; you breathe the same air now and help you get lost right now.

    Improving this can make sex purely magical.

2. **Emotional**

    Emotional tantric sex generally refers to a deep recall of love thoughts and the "worship" of another person's divinity. This means that you need to create an emotional connection with the bed. Here's how you can work on it:

    - **Try to Say What You Want to Do**

        No, you don't have to do this when you are in bed and having sex, but you can talk about it during dinner and the like. Sometimes it's important to tell your partner what's going on - for example, the sexual fantasies you've always had - so that he/she can also think about how to implement them. Make sure it's a two-way street: learn how to give in to your partner's needs.

- Recognize your emotional experiences with your partner.

Remember how you feel when you realize how much you love your partner. Try to delve into the deepest parts of the heart and find out what you really think about this person. Intimacy is not only about what you can physically share, but also how you know each other by heart.

- Remember that none of you is perfect.

Sometimes you expect so much from your partner that you forget that he/she can fulfill your wishes only if you communicate properly. Make your expectations come true, and I don't want something you know you can't give. Always work to improve the communication skills and dynamics that both of you have.

- Look into your eyes.

    To be aware of a strong emotional connection, it is important to learn to look into each other's eyes during sexual intercourse. As you progress, you'll notice how different you feel about your partner compared to normal or normal sex.

- Try to evaluate what you think about your partner in a sexual context.

    Are you delighted with the intimacy with your partner? What do you want to do with him and how do you think intimacy would improve your long-term relationship?

3. **Spiritual**

Spiritual tantric sex generally means feeling like one, associated with a "Supreme Being" or "God." And finally, you have a spiritual component that many people consider to be one of the most important parts of tantric sex. You can make it work like this:

- Remember that sex is not just a relationship; it is a relationship between two people.

    In short, you both have to be involved in engaging in and achieving tantric sex. The powerful and ecstatic feelings that can be felt in the heart of a tantric sexual experience do not come from "forcing" an act or a deliberate attempt to manipulate another person.

It must be possible to connect two people who trust each other and keep in touch (no wordplay is intended).

- Go beyond self-absorption and narcissism.

Always treat your partner honestly. Sexuality begins when you both reach maturity that is not based on narcissism or makes you feel less than you should.

As a couple, you have a life together; it's important to recognize that this is the highest priority, even during sex.

- Get out of reality.

You don't need to think about all the problems you have in bed with your partner. Just think about the moment. Focus on leaving your problems outside your sexual experience. Basically, tantric sex can be a kind of meditation session if done correctly.

- Sex can be virtuous without prose.

    Sex can be pure without one of you who could be a thriller. This happens when you both agree on what you want to do - and how you want it to happen.

- Tantric sex is also a form of prayer.

    Why? Because it evokes the deepest parts of your soul and helps you keep in touch with another person. When you pray, it's not just about wishing what is good for you; he also cares about others and sex should be like that.

In addition to mystical and cosmic experiences, most tantric masters also seek deeper and more personal experiences with other people and the world in which they live. They believe that if there is a deep connection, then space previously seen between two people will be replaced by the light of the Supreme Being. They believe that this spiritual presence activates etheric energy between two people, "connecting them together" so that they can become one.

They believe that Tantra is actually a divine path that should be practiced with the greatest divinity and holiness. Tantra should be practiced as if one was engaged in a spiritual "ritual," and like most spiritual worship, it is inevitable to honor and recognize the Supreme Being. However, in this ideology, when you practice tantric sex, the deity is actually contained in your partner instead of a vague picture.

Tantra is never an abstract form of sacred or sacred practice, but it is actually a practice in which experience with the Supreme Being is sent to the deepest areas of your senses. This does not mean, however, that you may not practice all other forms of worship or spirituality. The challenge of Tantra for all lovers is to feel, see, and hear the presence of the Supreme Being when they are united as one during tantric pranks.

Myths and the Truths about Tantric Sex and Tantra

Tantra is about celebrating sexuality and sensuality. It is a general misunderstanding that Tantra is based on sex. People, not fully aware of Tantra, know it from criticism.

Myth # 1: Tantric sex is about sex.

The truth: Tantric sex includes sex, but it's not just about genital contact. Tantric sex is about uniting souls, not just bodies. Genital contact or sex will only help increase the connection between souls. However, this is only possible if the couple feels at ease and are ready for this level of intimacy. Tantric sex includes various aspects that have absolutely nothing to do with sex.

Myth # 2: If you start practicing Tantra, you will simply give up pleasure.

The truth: This myth is loosely based on the previous myth. It's just a myth. Teaching Tantra does not include giving up sexual pleasure, as some yoga practices do. Tantra simply improves the level of pleasure. Tantric sex theory does not say that you must deny your desires. In fact, tantric sex encourages you to express your sexual desires freely. You don't have to imitate a yogi, sit cross-legged, or meditate for centuries to establish a connection with the Cosmos. Tantra realizes the importance of sex in the life of an individual and helps to use the undeveloped sexual energy present in the body to achieve happiness.

Myth # 3: Tantric sex increases sexual appetite and the need for pleasure that leads to business.

The truth: Tantric sex does not increase your sexual appetite and does not deceive you in the search for pleasure. Instead, it will help you control your desires and also help direct the sexual energy present in your body to a higher goal. Perhaps you were not even aware of your true potential. Tantric sex does not encourage having sex with multiple partners. This assumption has somehow reached many minds and is false.

Myth # 4: Turn you into a nymphomaniac.

The truth: Well, that's not true and it's pretty silly. Tantric sex helps to release all sexual energy present in the body, and also allows you to express yourself as easily as possible, but this does not mean that it will turn you into a nymphomaniac. However, the chances are that it will be misused. By exercising, you can control your desires and stop enjoying meaningless sex.

These common myths have spoiled the picture of tantric sex in the minds of the general public. This is not a taboo and should be practiced freely if you so choose.

CHAPTER 5:

Yantra

Yantra, in its literal translation from Sanskrit, means 'instrument' or a 'support.' In tantra practice, a Yantra is usually a geometrical design that is employed as a very effective tool to support the practitioner in meditative, contemplative, and concentration activities. Yantras represent the macrocosm in a microcosmic frame and acts as a gateway to and from the higher planes of consciousness. Yantras are all spiritually significant designs and every aspect has specific meanings pertaining to the higher planes of consciousness.

The Yantra in tantric practices behaves like a window to the universal divine being or the absolute one, as this power is many times referred to. When you compel your mind to focus on a single design or object (the yantra in this case), the overwhelming mental chatter that clutters your mind is reduced. With practice, it is possible to eliminate mindless chatter in your mind completely. When the mind has achieved calmness and complete stillness, the yantra is dropped by the practitioners. A seasoned tantric practitioner only needs to visualize the yantra in his mind to reach a calm state of mind.

Yantras are usually designed symmetrically in such a way that the practitioner's eyes can be focused on the center. Yantras can be drawn on paper, on wood, on metal, or directly on the earth. They can also be three-dimensional objects. In India, the most famous one is the Sri Vidya yantra that represents the deity Tripura Sundari. This symbol is a microcosm of the entire universe and is used to remind the practitioners that there is no difference between the object and the subject.

Operation of Yantras

'Form energy' of 'shape energy' or the concept that every form or shape emits a particular energy pattern and frequency, is the basis of the operation of any yantra. Examples of such yantras that are seen even in Judaism and Christianity include the 5-pointed star or the Pentagon, the Star of David, the pyramids, the Cross, etc. These shapes are given different degrees of negative and positive power (or evil and good power). In Tantra practices, only those shapes that have positive attributes, and those with harmonious and beneficial energies are used.

When a practitioner focuses on the particular yantra, his or her mind automatically tunes in to the 'resonating' frequency or energy pattern of that yantra. Continued focus helps in maintaining and amplifying this resonating effect. It is important to remember that the energy itself as a result of the focusing exercise comes from the macrocosm and not from the yantra.

Therefore, yantras are instruments or tools that help us achieve resonance with a particular frequency from the macrocosm. The yantra facilitates the practitioner to 'tune in' to the desired frequency from the cosmos. It is possible to effectively use yantras to put the practitioner into elevated energy levels in the universe.

Types of Yantras Used in Tantric Practices

Unfortunately, the Western world is yet to understand the true meaning and the resonating power of a yantra. Many dubious tantric schools claim that they can draw Yantras by drawing on their imagination. This is not true. Every emotion has a specific yantra associated with it through the energy that its form and shape represent.

The traditional Yantras were not drawn from imagination but revealed through divine design and clairvoyance. Showing a new yantra to the world requires the limitless tantric powers of a true guru. Taking all and sundry 'designs' available on the internet as a yantra will only reduce the powerful influence of your tantric practice.

Yantras and mantras are connected because a particular yantra needs to be focused on by chanting a corresponding mantra. Here are a few yantras, along with a basic understanding of each of their resonance.

- The Dot or the Bindu – The Bindu represented focalized energy brought on by intense concentration. It can be seen as a deposit or reservoir of concentrated energy. In Tantric practice, the dot is considered to represent Siva Himself, the masculine source of all creation.

- The Triangle or the Trikona – This is a symbol of Shakti, the feminine source of all creation. A downward-pointing triangle represents the female sexual organ, the yoni, the Universe's supreme source. An upward-pointing triangle represents the supreme spiritual aspiration of being one with the absolute. Also, the downward triangle represents water which tends to flow down while the upward triangle represents fire which goes up always.

- The 6-Pointed Star of the Shatkona – Two triangles, one upward-facing, and the other downward-facing, superimposed over each other combine to form the shatkona, referred to as David's star in Judaism. This symbol represents the union of Siva and Shakti, without which there can be no creation.

- The Circle or the Chakra – Representing rotation, the circle is another commonly used symbol either by itself or as part of a more complex yantra in tantric practices. The process is also a very closely connected movement with spiraling movement, based on the evolution in the macrocosm. Moreover, the chakra or the circle is also a representation of the creative void and perfection. It symbolizes the wind element of nature.

- The Lotus Symbol – This is a symbol of variety (each petal is representing something different) and purity owing to the flower's ability to rise above a dirty pond to remain beautiful and pure.

- The Square or the Bhupura – Representing the element earth, the square symbol is usually the external contour of a yantra. Usually, a yantra uses the square as the contour and the dot as the center. This is the concept in tantra that the universe starts from the subtle (the dot – concentrated energy) and moves toward the gross (or the earth and life systems).

Many of the complex yantras also include other symbols such as arrows, swords, tridents, etc., representing the direction and purpose of the action of the form energy the yantra signifies.

How to Use Yantras in Tantric Practices

As already explained, resonance is the critical aspect of any yantra. The resonating effect of the yantra can be initiated and maintained by focusing on its image. The mind should be tuned to the resonating energy of the particular yantra for activation and sustenance of energy flow.

Here are some instructions on the correct use of yantras:

- Hang the Yantra on any wall facing east or north ensuring the center of the image is in line with your eyes.
- When meditating, sit in a comfortable position that you are accustomed to.
- Inhale through the nose and exhale through your mouth in your natural breathing rhythm without trying to control your breath.
- Focus on the center of the yantra with as little blinking as possible. Keep the focus of your eyes on the center and watch the entire yantra as one.
- You can start with 5 minutes each day of this meditating exercise and then slowly increase the duration until you can do about half an hour a day.
- It is recommended that you aspire to achieve the levels of resonating energy that the yantra can deliver and your aspiration is bound to be fulfilled sooner than later.
- Seasoned tantric practitioners can reach such amazing depths in their focus that it is difficult for them to tell whether the yantra is within them or whether they are inside the yantra.

CHAPTER 6:

Mantra

With profound practices like yoga and contemplation winding up progressively prevalent, it appears as though everybody is discussing mantras. Be that as it may, what precisely is a mantra, and how are you expected to utilize it?

In our westernized, cutting edge otherworldly rehearses, "mantra" has progressed toward becoming as standard as "goal." But the two are entirely different.

The word mantra can be stalled into two sections: "man," which means mind, and "tra," which means transport or vehicle. As such, a mantra is an instrument of the psyche — a groundbreaking sound or vibration that you can use to enter a secret government of reflection.

Like a seed planted with the goal of blooming into a beautiful lasting, a mantra can be thought of as a seed for invigorating an aim.

Yoga and Mantra

This mantra is utilized in quiet reiteration during development to help keep the mind centered. It has been said that in yoga, Asanas are stances of the body and mantras are stances of the brain. Mantras, when utilized in this design, are progressively similar to confirmations and help to keep you associated with a specific perspective.

Sanskrit and Mantra

Getting to the old foundation, all things considered, mantra, at its center, is the premise of every single religious custom, sacred texts, and petitions. At the point when deliberately picked and utilized quietly, mantras are said to be able to help adjust your intuitive driving forces, propensities, and burdens. Mantras, when spoken or recited, direct the mending intensity of Prana (life power vitality) and, in conventional Vedic practices, can be utilized to empower and get to otherworldly conditions of cognizance. As a profound practice, Mantra ought to be done all the time for a while for its ideal impacts to occur.

Toward the day's end, the mantra is intended to take you back to effortlessness. We live in such an unpredictable world that it is anything but difficult to lose all sense of direction in every one of the subtleties. Mantras can enable you to hover back to the oversimplified way to deal with life and spotlight those things that motivate you and satisfy you.

Reflection and Mantra

In this unique circumstance, mindfulness alludes to the capacity to focus on the decisions you make in your regular daily existence and perceive when something is not working so you can transform it. Numerous individuals face a great deal of pressure every day. Before the part of the bargain, prepared to crash. At that point, you rehash the cycle the following day.

Building up a day-by-day contemplation practice causes you to develop an increasingly present, quiet, and adjusted lifestyle, which swells out into each other part of your life. Mantras can help take you back to that current situation with the psyche.

You've most likely heard the word mantra previously. Be that as it may, what you can be sure of is this is an otherworldly practice, and it is as old as it is significant.

We will investigate what mantras are, the different ways they can be utilized, and best of all — how you can give them something to do in your very own life for mind-blowing mending, strengthening, and change.

All in all, what is a mantra? It is a word, sound, syllable, or expression that has an incredible vibration reverberation.

They are utilized in reflection, yoga, and in the otherworldly practices of Buddhism, Hinduism, and Jainism.

You can utilize a mantra to think about your vitality, open your chakras, and build up your mystic mindfulness. Otherworldly expressions, when opened, can raise your awareness. This training is so convincing and powerful. You have no clue where it could take you.

Personal mantra?

An individual mantra is an explanation that spurs and motivates you to be your best self.

With a personal mantra, you confirm how you need to carry on with your life. Also, it can help propel you to finish your objectives, both actually and expertly.

What Is Mantra Healing?

It has been demonstrated that reciting, music, and mantras strongly affect our cerebrum.

Mantras are fiery sound equations that moderate us down and permit us to see everything unmistakably. They give us a point of view.

Reciting quiets, the body and actuates various normal substantial capacities and procedures. It can likewise help in mending the psyche and body from addictions, such as smoking or liquor. Also, reciting can reinforce the resistant framework.

Reciting can lower pulse, lessen feelings of anxiety, increment hormone level execution, and abate nervousness and gloom.

Who might have imagined that this straightforward practice could have such control?

Yoga and Om Shanti

Om Shanti is maybe one of the most notable and open mantras utilized today. If you've at any point gone to a yoga class, odds are you've heard it.

All in all, what does Om Shanti mean? Indeed, there is a very immediate interpretation of Om Shanti. Om is not to such an extent as a word as it is a sound, an inclination, and a positive reverberation.

Om is said to be the sound of the universe. This single syllable incorporates the cycle of death and resurrection. Reciting the word Om carries you into an enthusiastic arrangement with the universe.

Anyway, shouldn't something be said about Shanti? Shanti is a Sanskrit word that signifies, "Harmony." Together, the Om Shanti importance is intended to pass on: Universal Peace.

It is regularly utilized as a welcome in yoga as a method for recognizing a kindred expert and wishing them harmony.

The absolute first mantras were utilized by Hindus in quite a while more than 3,000 years prior. A few hundred years after the fact, after Buddhism started to prosper, mantras began to be joined into their otherworldly practice as well.

Buddhist mantras depend on the heavenly lessons of the Buddha and the bodhisattvas. Here are three conventional Buddhist mantras you probably will not have known about previously:

- "Om Mani Padme Hum"

    This mantra is utilized in Tibetan Buddhism. That is to say, "I currently conjure the Universal sound, the gem, the objective of Enlightenment, love, and sympathy, Lotus shrewdness, and an unadulterated unified solidarity of insight with training."

    This is a routine with regards to empathy. It is utilized to look for and spread compassion for oneself as well as other people.

- "Om Muni Mahamuni Shakyamuniye Svaha"

    This signifies, "I summon the universal sound, Buddha-nature and the shrewd one, insightful one of the Shakyans, hail to thee!"

- "Om Vasudhare Svaha"

    Additionally, called the Buddhist cash mantra, it is utilized as a supplication to the bodhisattva of earth and wealth, Vasudhara. In Buddhism, Vasudhara is believed to exemplify the female soul and is the partner to the Hindu goddess, Lakshmi.

Reflection mantras are a great method to build your care during contemplation. They serve as a point of convergence for your consideration, a similar way you may utilize a light, a photograph, or a statue.

There are many contemplation mantras you can access for nothing.

The best part? They go about as a type of guided contemplation to enable you to remain grounded and present.

Here is a couple to kick you off:

- "Ham-Sah." Or, "I am that." This aide advises us that we are onlookers and separate from our human encounters and enduring.

- "Aham Prema." Or, "I am Divine Love."

- "Om Shanti, Shanti, Shanti." Or, "Genuine feelings of serenity, body, and discourse."

- "Om Tat Sat." Or, "All that is."

By what means can a mantra best be utilized?

Anyway, how would you utilize a reflection mantra? When you've chosen one, you'd like to attempt, locate a peaceful spot to start your contemplation practice.

When you are prepared, set the goal for your reflection. This is the place your chosen mantra will truly sparkle. Regardless of whether you'd like to ruminate for better wellbeing, more stillness, or only for a snapshot of harmony, set that aim before you start.

When you are prepared, start your mantra. You can say it so anyone can hear or in your mind.

Keep in mind; it is anything but a race. You can say it the same number or as multiple times as you'd like. Perhaps you have a specific number as a primary concern. Perhaps not. Essentially rehash your mantra gradually and with a goal.

Consider what your picked mantra implies. Harp on the individual words. Let the reverberation and vibration of every syllable ring.

This type of reflective practice is a ground-breaking one. Regardless of whether you've never attempted it, you will undoubtedly encounter transformative outcomes. Try it out.

Presently, in light of the fact that mantras are a 3,000 years-old profound practice doesn't mean they aren't similarly as viable today as they were in those days!

Mantras have changed throughout the years to oblige our cutting-edge frames of mind and recognitions.

A mantra shouldn't be articulated in Sanskrit to hold control. A mantra simply should be something that impacts you on a significant and individual level.

Mantras are frequently utilized in contemplation as an approach to remain engaged and focused. Be that as it may, you can utilize mantras from multiple points of view.

Print one out to set up on your divider. Record one on the network board at work. Slip a post-its mantra into your companion's handbag for an additional portion of motivation.

CHAPTER 7:

Yin & Yang

When you begin to follow the path of tantric sex, you begin to find a change in yourself. You find yourself changing how you view yourself and how you view the world. You find yourself looking at relationships that will last a lifetime. Through your journey, you will learn that every man and woman has a certain level of divinity in them. You will start to view sex as a sacred act instead of just a physical act. You will also learn to love deeper and find that you are soaring to different levels of bliss.

You will only have a successful journey when you relieve yourself from any preconceived notions. You should not think of what you need to do and what your lover must do to please you.

You will learn the basic concepts of tantric sex and identify new exciting ways to live and love. The Yin and the Yang: Which is male and which is female?

You must be familiar with the stereotypes that men are from Mars, and women are from Venus. This implies that men are assertive and extremely powerful, while women are soft and fragile, who are only fit for nurturing. There are other stereotypes that men do not show any feelings whatsoever, while women have a plethora of emotion that is ready to unleash itself in a second. It has also been said that women do not take credit for the work that they do, since being outgoing is something only men are familiar with. Over the last few years, there has been a drastic change in the way men and women think.

Tantric sex is a firm follower of the fact that men and women do have opposite characteristics. This is the elementary principle of the Tantra. The eastern theories claim that Yin represents feminism, while Yang represents masculinity. But there is no concrete proof that a woman cannot have Yang characteristics or that a man cannot have Yin characteristics. Rather than viewing men and woman as two entities, you should begin to focus on the energies. The Tantra believes in the amalgamation of these two energies.

Shiva and Shakti

The most common image of the Yin and the Yang is the Hindu divine couple Lord Shiva and Goddess Shakti. Lord Shiva represents the entire universe since he is considered the creator, and Goddess Shakti represents the root of all energy. The union of the two deities creates a longing in you and every other human being to be treated like a god or a goddess.

The male energy that is found in Lord Shiva represents ecstasy, while the energy in Goddess Shakti represents wisdom. This magical combination is what helps a person attain enlightenment. This perfect couple is always represented in numerous entwined positions – either dancing or embracing or standing together. There are other positions where Goddess Shakti is wrapped around Lord Shiva, with her legs propped around his hips. The dancing position by far is the most sacred since they can free their spirit, giving them a chance to attain enlightenment.

Understanding the Opposites

You may have made divisions amongst you and your partner. You first have to identify and understand these divisions to strike a balance between the opposite energies. There are quite a few stereotypical characteristics that you may relate to. You will have to identify those characteristics and make a note of them. You have to go from one extreme to the next. You should ask your partner to do this too. You will then have to see how you can embrace the extreme characteristics that you and your partner have. You have to identify how you can strike a balance between the polarities that exist between you and your partner. You will have to identify the Yin to your partner's Yang and vice versa.

You might now wonder if it is true that opposites attract. Sit back and think for yourself. You will be able to answer this question on your own. Try analyzing your past relationships. See how you and your partner were different from each other. Identify whether the differences were complemented by each other. This will help you analyze your future relationships as well.

My Partner is My Beloved

Tantra is not mad love but sacred love. You are honoring your partner and cherishing your partner while making love. You will shower unconditional love with your partner. When you are talking to your partner, use loving words like 'darling' or 'beloved'. You will find that those little words have aroused feelings of love within your partner. Call your partner with the aforementioned loving words when talking about him or her in public. You might find it strange to do so, but you will be sending out a message of love to the person you are speaking to.

The Desire Spectrum

You will find yourself with new views of desire. You may feel a desire every time you think of someone. You may comment on how you want a guy or how hot a girl is when you see them passing. You only feel these desires when you feel incomplete. Since you feel incomplete, you always want another person. You find yourself feeling needy and feeling wanted. But when you do get the person you want; you begin to want something more. You want someone prettier, more interesting, and sometimes someone richer. Through tantric sex, you will be able to detach yourself from superficial needs. This will help you create a healthier relationship with your partner.

You Feel Empowered to Say What You Want!

When you find yourself empowered, you can set boundaries both during sex and in life in general. You find yourself with a new level of self – esteem. In tantric sex, you own your body and your soul. When your partner wants you to enter you, he must ask for your permission. You should not be afraid and have to say yes or no as the situation demands. You have to stop and say that you do not want to be touched in a way that is not comfortable with it. You empower your partner when you speak the truth this way. You will be giving your partner the methods to use to please you. You have to be okay with how you are touched and how you feel.

CHAPTER 8:

Tantric Communication

Does your associate virtually recognize how you want to be touched? How do you want to be loved? Imagine you may get precisely what you need in a mattress.

Before I knew approximately Tantra, I spent many a time mendacity with inside the fingers of my lover wishing he might do that or that. Thinking that if handiest he did this, then matters might be a lot higher for me. Conversely, I discovered myself questioning if he virtually favored what I gave to him if I turned into pleasurable his sexual and sensual goals. Obviously, the verbal exchange channels had been now no longer in particular open, subsequently we each wasted a whole lot of time questioning approximately the opposite's goals and wishes.

If we don't inform every different what we need and like, how are we able to in all likelihood anticipate our associate to satisfy our maximum mystery wishes intuitively?

Information Gathering in Tantra, one-of-a-kind strategies is used to open the verbal exchange channels and to create verbal intimacy in a context of considering. Being heard and listened to is as vital as sharing and telling our reality.

A Tantric verbal exchange starts off evolved with developing a sacred area. Sit down throughout from every different and proportion an include. Give every different compliment, bow right all the way down to your associate. With this exercise you're integrating a tantric mini-ritual into your lifestyles, making the verbal exchange exercise a unique occasion to be commemorated and cherished.

Now set parameters for the exercise. For instance, one character speaks, at the same time as the opposite listens for an agreed length of time, say ten mins. After the 10 mins, transfer roles.

The verbal exchange exercise usually revolves around a query. You could make up any query. For instance, "How do you want to be touched?" The speaker will reply to the query spontaneously. The listener will ask the query after which pay attention. If your associate runs out of answers, ask the identical query again. Note that this isn't a workout in communique approximately the subject, however, an excursion to benefit records approximately the opposite character and to exercise the artwork of listening.

The listener's function is to pay attention without a schedule and take with inside the records. By schedule, I suggest this – believe your lover tells you that she would love you to stroke her breasts in a total one-of-a-kind manner than you've got been doing when you consider that you acquire collectively. If you had a schedule at the same time as listening, you would possibly listen to yourself thinking, "How come she by no means instructed me this earlier than? Am I a total failure? Am I now no longer proper sufficient for her? Is she going to go away from me due to the fact I can't deliver her what she needs?"

If you had no schedule at the same time as listening, you'll take the records in and keep with the tantric exercise. And at the subsequent opportunity, you would possibly try and contact her breasts inside the manner she described. And you'll be pleasantly amazed at the aid of using her reaction!

At the quilt of the exercise, proportion an include and thank every different for generously imparting this treasured record.

In this Tantric verbal exchange, we discover ways to consider that the opposite character will deliver us what we really need due to the fact we created a secure and sacred area to invite for it

You might also additionally experience awkward answering an intimate query. Dare to speak! You are expressing yourself to your associate who desires to recognize all approximately you. Although awkwardness and shyness are a part of lifestyles, strive for something one-of-a-kind. For instance, you and your associate may describe how you want to be touched in very erotic terms. Or you may strive for the use of poetic language. This is one-of-a-kind out of your daily terminology. The humor and a laugh concerned creates a detail of lightheartedness that makes it clean to each specific goal and pays attention to them.

Loving feedback, another thing about Tantric verbal exchange, is the sensitive artwork of feedback. Imagine you're on a mattress together along with your lover and you're stroking his muscular shoulders. You suppose which you are doing a lovely activity and that he likes it very much. He lies there wishing you'll rub his shoulders harder. He receives bored stiff and all of a sudden informs you, "No, that's now no longer proper, rub my shoulders difficult as opposed to doing those feather-mild strokes." You at once flinch and don't need to head-on. You suppose you're now no longer proper sufficient that he doesn't like what you're doing.

Now believe this. He says delicately, "That felt very proper, my lovely beloved, however proper now I might pick a hint that may be a little bit firmer." You will experience mollified, preferred, and demonstrated for what you've got been doing, and can be handiest too glad to oblige and deliver him what he requests.

This is a great instance of tantric verbal exchange. Validate the one that you love earlier than you ask for something one-of-a-kind. Offer love and appreciation – she or he turned into doing his or her quality, after all – after which inform her or him what she or he should do to thrill you even greater.

Steve and I are surprised at what number of new matters we discover approximately every different in those verbal exchange rituals. We ought to have requested the identical query one hundred instances, and whenever the records we acquire from every different is one-of-a-kind and new. This is recuperation for each people and brings us nearer collectively.

Tantra is an effective transformational device this is a lot greater than intercourse!

There is a cultural craving for greater connection and intimacy in relationships. There is likewise a name for sacred and religious connections. People of all ages, genders, and sexual orientations are feeling the want for an area to connect to their frame, mind, and spirit in the community. Tantra gives methods to deepen your dating with yourself and others.

For people who are new to Tantra, it's far an exercise that mixes movement, breath, meditation, bodywork, and sound to help the powerful machine inside the frame, additionally called chakras, to open. This commencing lets in dormant power, additionally called kundalini, to transport up from the pelvis, alongside the spine. As this lifestyles-pressure power actions up the spine, it allows one to convert and heal. The recuperation includes loosening constrictions inside the frame that broadens for the duration of lifestyles. When the constrictions are loosened, one's real identity is revealed. Transformation takes vicinity, in addition to lifestyle shifts: sizeable bodily and emotional fitness improvements, new jobs, new or deeper partnerships, actions to one's dream location — those are simply a number of the results I actually have witnessed.

The goal of tantric practices is to increase one's frame and enjoy returned to the soul's authentic essence (called Purusha in Sanskrit): who you had been as a fetus, freed from strain or trauma, and who you're developing into as you end up unfastened. This is whilst we will come into our fullest potential, with acute attention and clean, loving reference to others.

On my very own Tantra path, and as a practitioner, I actually have held the area for lots to increase into their fullest selves. Over and over, I actually have visible that after chakras open, feelings stir. After all, they have become blocked or shriveled due to the fact one turned into now no longer covered or did now no longer experience secure being oneself. Contractions can end result now no longer handiest from a twist of fate or abuse, however additionally, from the consistent messages we acquire from society to be a person we're now no longer. Contractions inside the frame are an herbal reaction to shield your soul, which needs a lot to be unfastened to specific itself. However, the contractions have an effect on our cap potential to create and to permit pass of unsupportive habits, and additionally how we connect to others.

Inviting the chakra machine to open calls for braveness and readiness to take that leap, trusting that you may be supported and guarded as you heal and open to residing your real destiny.

Why are such a lot of humans turning to Tantra to clear up their dating challenges?

Tantra gives easy, beneficial verbal exchange strategies you could exercise and use at once for your everyday lives. Tantra can end up your new manner of relating — with a goal, care, and passion. We assist our college students to be sincere approximately what they revel in and what they don't in any given second.

Sexual abuse survivors and people with different sexual issues discover Tantra to be recuperation. We all want a discussion board to talk about sexual issues brazenly without shame and an area to research new methods of connecting in detail which are sacred, a laugh, and exciting.

Today, with the multiplied use of era for verbal exchange, each companion frequently retaining down complete-time jobs, and they want to coordinate parenting schedules, couples frequently glide apart. Tantra assists you in connecting, igniting a new passion, and considering why you got here collectively to proportion your lives.

Tantra-primarily based practices totally, just like the Divine Love Meditation below, assist domesticate intimacy with oneself and others.

Divine Love Meditation

Try working towards this meditation regularly, and word in case your verbal exchange transforms to a greater loving form — also, word how this fashion of verbal exchange impacts your relationships with others.

Tantra is ready to turn into embodied. Obviously, if you're analyzing this, you're embodied; you manifested in the world as a frame that homes your spirit. However, to be truly "embodied" to have intentional heightened attention to our very own presence. The frame is a doorway via which we will step into a fair extra experience of ourselves. By centering inside the frame, we open ourselves to what's past the frame, to a better vibration of our very own existence.

Some religious training takes an "out-of-frame" technique. Tantra rather invitations us to end up absolutely gift in the frame, to get entry to the deeper, non-bodily reality of who we're. It isn't approximately being greater bodily. It is ready centering ourselves with inside the remaining right here and now of our being.

How does this observe verbal exchange? Well, you recognize the expression "speak me heads?" It is used to explain TV pundits who're usually giving us their limitless opinions. In an experience, we're all "speak my heads." We speak from our heads. "I suppose, consequently I am," asserted Descartes returned with inside the sixteenth century. Identifying with our mind is certainly a not unusual place of self-referencing, of spotting who we're. Yet is it sufficient?

Thoughts are treasured and deliver a path to our lives. Emotions are an aggregate of our intellectual mind and the sensations or emotions we enjoy thru our frame. How mind experience in our bodies, what physical sensations we enjoy whilst we suppose or specific our very own or listen to any other's mind, and wherein we experience them, can deliver us effective clues to our internal reality. Thoughts and frame emotions feed on every different, impact every different. Thoughts generate emotions. Sensations that we enjoy with inside the frame cause mind.

CHAPTER 9:

Tantric Massage and Tantric Yoga

Massage is defined as a succession of strokes performed to promote muscular relaxation. However, tantric massage is more than that. The tantric touch stimulates, nurtures, and heals the body, the mind, the emotions, and the spirit.

When done on its own, tantric massage can be an erotic experience. It can also turn into a therapeutic journey. When done before sex, tantric massage is a means of prolonging and building pleasure. When used as foreplay, the tantric touch relaxes your mind and your body so it becomes more receptive to your partner's gifts. It enables your sexual arousal to mount before it reaches its pinnacle. This way, your orgasms can become longer and more intense.

Tantric sex is safe and healthy lovemaking. Some couples may feel pressured to engage in an intercourse in the early dating phase before they're emotionally attached or psychologically prepared. Using tantric massage as a pleasurable alternative for intercourse relieves them of this pressure. Tantric massage can be a fun and sexy way of getting to know each other deeper so that you'll have ample time to connect with each other emotionally. This way, once you finally decide to have sex, it becomes more meaningful and more satisfying.

Benefits of Tantric Massage

The busy and hectic life that we lead these days affects both men and women, and it causes several physicals, emotional, and even sexual disorders. Stress doesn't discriminate, and it could trouble a person belonging to any age group, sex, or age. People need some relief if they want to enjoy their life to the fullest and they also have to replenish their strength to keep up with their hectic lifestyle. Massage can help in providing much-needed comfort and help you relax. Among all the different types of massages that exist, tantric massage is gaining popularity. The main aim of a tantric massage is to provide you with a sensual experience that will also improve your health. Even though it is erotic, it helps the whole body to relax and has got several benefits.

- **Stress Buster**

    Tantric massage can help you clear your mind, make your body feel light and help you relax. You can let go of all the tension and stress. Therefore, a session of tantric massage is recommended whenever you feel stressed. Stress is capable of making you feel miserable. If it isn't handled properly, it can cause several health problems as well.

- **Sex Education**

    In many cultures around the world, sex education isn't adequate, and this leaves both genders unprepared for any sexual interaction or even sensuality. A tantric massage is the best way in which you can learn about your body. It provides you with a serial interaction that will help you to understand how your body works. It provides you with an insight into how your body works and the different parts that will make you feel other sensations. When you interact with your partner, it will be helpful to know what excites and pleases you both.

- **Premature Ejaculation**

    Premature ejaculation usually tends to occur due to the pressure of performance. In most societies and cultures, men are considered to be the "doers," which puts an added pressure on them and causes them to ejaculate prematurely. Tantric massage helps in taking this pressure off them and lets them just enjoy the sexual act. When there isn't an expectation of them to perform well and without any specific goal in mind, men can perform well sexually. This will help in rectifying the problem of premature ejaculation.

    Tantric massage will help in teaching you to enjoy the moment, and during intercourse, it would also improve a man's ability to hold off his climax for a while longer. It is all about drawing out the pleasure to make the experience more intense.

- **Orgasm in Older Men**

As time passes by, and while the body starts aging, the body's hormone levels tend to decline and because of this older men feel little or even no sexual arousal, which means that they aren't capable of reaching an orgasm. Tantric massage can be beneficial for older men. This sensual massage helps in stimulating their senses and also helps in the production of the sex hormones and thereby helping them deal with problems like erectile dysfunction and the lack of achieving an orgasm.

- **Women and Sex**

In most cases, women don't enjoy intercourse. This could be caused due to various reasons ranging from their lover's inability to please them or even their lack of knowledge about their body. Women are sensual creatures, and it takes them a while longer to achieve an orgasm. Most might not even be aware of their bodies or what they like and dislike. Tantric massage will help them in understanding their bodies and their needs better. It will help them in deriving greater pleasure and even sensuality during any form of sexual activity.

Tantric massage helps in awakening your senses. It is sensual. We tend to perceive the world around us through our senses, and the awakening of the senses sharpens this perception of ours. Tantric massage is a therapeutic massage that has various health benefits. It can help relieve body pains and aches, stimulate your immune system, and increase your fertility. Many women can't orgasm, and tantric massage helps integrate your mind and body thereby facilitating their ability to reach an orgasm. Tantric massage tends to be empowering on various levels regardless of the characteristics of an individual. Tantric massage also provides the greatest form of relaxation and pleasure for your mind, body, and soul without having to reciprocate.

Tantric massage involves the massaging of all the parts of the body. Having one's genitals massaged is quite a fulfilling experience. It also helps in creating a conscious connection between all the areas of a person's life. A massage without any expectations is quite a liberating experience. Tantric massage helps let go of the illusion of separation that exists and remedies this divide in every individual's life. It can also pave the way for a full-body orgasm.

- **Tantric Yoga**

    Tantric yoga helps improve the nature of one's relationship and cherishes and imparts delicate exercise to accomplices. It is an easy-to-execute yoga routine for sex accomplices to build the progression of sex yielding energy. It additionally helps in standard practice for making your body resistible, with a decent body, personality, and soul both inside and outside the room.

- **Straightforward Yoga Movements**

    This segment will enable you to get familiar with a couple of fundamental yoga represents that you can perform to improve your general wellbeing and stamina. In the following segment, you will learn about the diverse tantric activities you can, and your accomplices can perform together. This will help in expanding your closeness and solace level with each other.

    - **The Head Lift**

        Ensure that you are standing up straight for this. At that point tilt your head upward, what's more, tilt it in such a way, that string from the sky was pulling it upwards. Keep your mouth shut, and you should breathe in through your nose. When you are breathing in, ensure that you are moving your shoulder bones in reverse to appear that they are attempting to contact one another. It should feel like your feet are fixed to the ground. Loosen up your position and afterward rehash this procedure.

- **The Cobra Postures**

   You can rest on the floor or a yoga tangle. Presently stretch out your body to make sure that your stomach is contacting the floor. At that point place your hands under your bears with the goal that your elbows are set at the back. Lift your chest off the floor also, tilt your head with the goal that it would seem that a bend. Ensure that you are looking upwards. This posture should like a cobra that is going to strike. Loosen up your position and after that recurrent this procedure.

- **The Cat Postures**

   When you are finished with the Cobra present, you should delicately bring down your head furthermore, gradually ascend on your knees. This should appear as though you are squatting, so stretch your spine the other way than what you did in the Cobra present.

- **The Resting Postures**

    When you have completed the Cat present, you should expect the Cobra present. Stretch your arms outwards. Take in profoundly and unreservedly. Ensure that your temple is lying on the ground and that your chest is contacting your knees.

- **Tantric Exercises**

    If you need to add some use to your routine with regards to Tantric sex, at that point, you can start rehearsing a couple of activities and breathing procedures that will help you in making your sexual experience far and away superior. Just as relaxing systems, these activities are most appropriate when finished with your accomplice, yet they should be possible on your own also. These activities and breathing systems have been referenced in this segment.

- **Shoulder Stand**

    Shoulder stands are useful for ladies for accepting the different Tantric stances effortlessly, yet on the other hand, men can rehearse them also. For playing out a basic shoulder represent, the individual should rest level on a tangle or even the floor with his/her legs extended straight and their hands resting close by. At that point, the individual will need to lift the legs at a 90-degree edge to achieve their upper-middle stay stuck to the floor. Their legs ought to be lifted somewhat higher than their lower back, and their hands ought to be put on their back for supporting this pose. Rehearsing this strategy will help in building up the truly necessary adaptability for accepting different Tantric sex positions.

- **Boat Posture**

This posture is by and by supportive for ladies. The individual playing out this posture ought to sit with a straight back, and their legs ought to be loosened up. At that point, the individual should lift their legs at a 45-degree end and, after that, stretch their hands outwards with the goal that their fingers are pointing towards their feet. Attempt and keep up this posture for three minutes and after that, unwind. Rehash this posture multiple times.

- **Three-Legged Pooch Posture**

    This posture is useful for extending the hamstring muscles, and these are very regularly utilized in Tantric sex. For playing out, this represents, the individual must lie down on their stomach on a tangle while their hands are set on their sides. Your palms ought to be placed alongside the chest and bolster your feet with your toes. Lift your body in such a way that your toes maintain your body weight. This position ought to appear as though your body is making a triangle, with the floor framing the triangle's base. The correct leg should then be gradually lifted upwards. Lift your leg to the extent your body would allow. At that point, come back to a nonpartisan position and rehash the equivalent with the other leg.

- **Extension Posture**

    This is a representation that is appropriate for both genders. For playing out this procedure, you should rest on your back, and, after that, twist your legs in such a way so your knees are pointing upwards.

Your feet ought to be set near your bum. The lower middle ought to be lifted, and your hands should lie on either side of your body for offering help. Rehash these multiple times.

CHAPTER 10:

Tantric Sex Positions

Right now, you will find out about various Tantric sex positions and procedures that you can use for spicing up your sexual coexistence.

The Sidewinder

This position is animated from a similar name's yoga position, and this procedure takes into account deep entrance. It likewise accommodates the couple to keep in touch. For playing out this method, the lady should rest on her side and support her chest area's heaviness with her hands' assistance. She should lift one of her legs and place it on her darling's shoulder while the other portion is lying on the bed. A variety of this equivalent position is that the man can rest behind the lady and enter his partner.

The Yab Yum

The Yab Yum position is viewed as probably the best situation for having tantric sex. It is a genuinely simple situation to perform, and it takes into consideration synchronous climaxes. This position helps in animating quite a few places. Likewise, the man's hands happen to be free right now, he can touch his darling's body however he sees fit, since the couple would confront one another, it takes into consideration enthusiastic kisses also. The man should sit leg over leg on the bed or some other agreeable surface and hold his back straight. The lady should straddle him and fold her legs over his lower back. It takes into account delayed here and there developments that can help the couple in accomplishing an all-around planned climax.

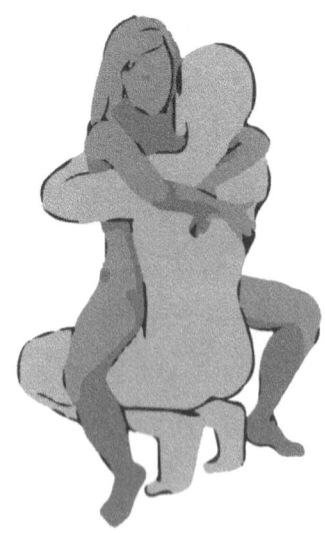

The Latch

This posture permits the man to get a decent see his sweetheart's face and the other way around. This is an extremely attractive posture and aids in pleasuring both partners. For playing out this procedure, the lady should be situated on a high stage like a table or even the kitchen counter. She will then need to recline and adjust her upper-middle and head with her hands' assistance by inclining onto her elbows. The man should remain between her separated legs and enter her. This represents that doesn't need to be limited to the room and is ideal for an off-the-cuff cavort.

The Butterfly

This method is accepted to allow both the partners to achieve a significant level of rapture and consider deep entrance. For playing out this system, the young lady should rest on the table so that her butt lies at the edge of the table. The man should help lift her lower back marginally off the table and afterward place both her legs over his shoulders. Her vagina would be free for him to infiltrate while remaining in the middle of her legs. Since her legs are shut together, this fixes the vaginal waterway and gives a tight fit. The man should enter her while her butt is in midair.

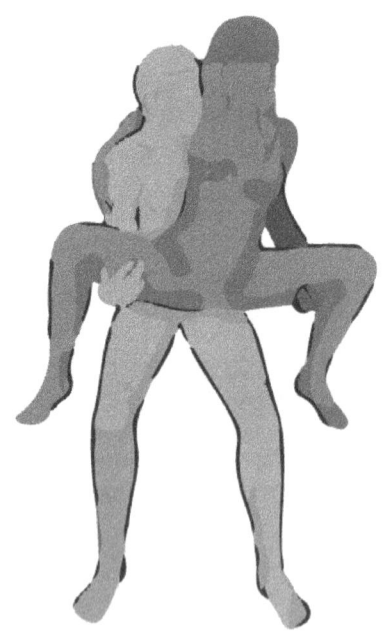

The Double Decker

This is an amazingly suggestive posture and will help in accomplishing a climax with no problem at all. The man will likewise be given a decent perspective on all the activity going on down there, and his hands will likewise have unlimited access to lay with his sweetheart's butt. This position is very enabling for ladies since they have all the control here. For playing out this system, the man should sit on the bed while his legs are collapsed under his body. The lady will then need to confront him and place her feet on either side of her darling while her feet are set level superficially to give her some help. When she has brought down herself onto his erect penis, she will just need to begin moving advances and reverse or even decide on a here and there movement. The man should kick back and have fun.

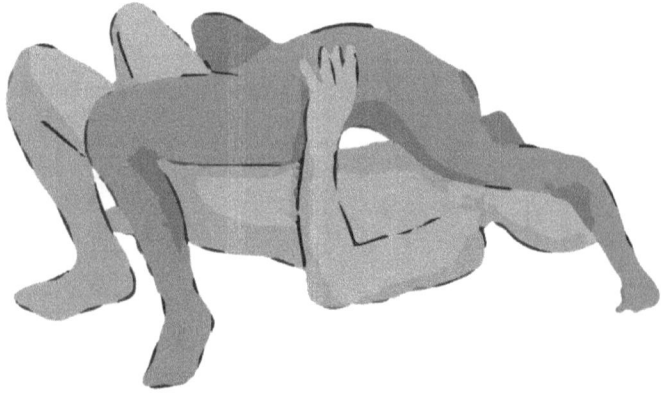

The Last Place Anyone Would Want to Be

This is an extraordinary posture since it permits both the gatherings to have a similar control measure and ooze a similar measure of pressure for having a great sexual encounter. People will have an equivalent balance right now. For playing out this represents, the man should sit on the bed and support his chest area with his knees. He will then need to move the lower portion of his legs in reverse and place them marginally separated. The lady will then need to expect a similar position. Yet, she will do as such while confronting ceaselessly from him and her run would be squeezing into his scrotum and her back against his chest. Her legs would be joined and afterward set in the space that is accessible between his legs and the man should enter her from behind. For this situation to be compelling, both the partners should remain as near to one another as could reasonably be expected.

Skiff

This position is a slight adjustment of the lady on top position. Right now, bodies should be situated so that both the partners will find a good pace great take a gander at one another's face while occupied with the demonstration. For playing out this, the man should sit down on a seat that can marginally twist in reverse. The lady will then need to put herself on his lap and place her legs on either side of the seat. The young lady should fire an allover development without anyone else. Her partner can help her by setting his hand under her bum and helping her move in an upwards and downwards way.

The Mermaid

This is a somewhat fluctuated adaptation of the butterfly, and it takes into consideration a more solace and better hold. Right now, a man can play with his darling's feet. Remember that feet are viewed as one of the most touchy and erogenous pieces of a lady's body. For playing out this method, the lady should expect a similar situation as she did in the butterfly, however, her butt ought to be propped with the assistance of a pad. Her legs should loosen up and ought to be at a 90-degree edge. The man should stand near the table and infiltrate her.

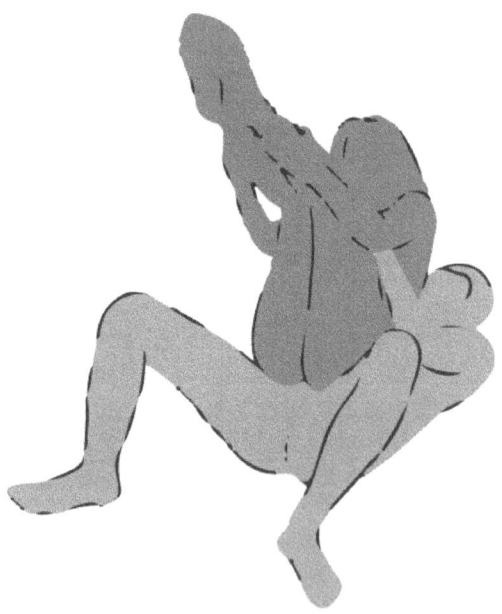

Tsunami

This posture is very agreeable, and it is a sensual treat. This will knock your socks off. This posture is a slight alteration of the exemplary minister style. Right now, a lady should expect the job that a man, as a rule, does in the teaching style. The man should rest level on his back for playing out this, and his arms should be put close by. The lady should lie over him, and the man should embed his penis into her vagina. The lady should loosen up her legs with the goal that they are resting on him. Her palms ought to be put on his lower arm for giving her some help. The lady will then need to begin moving her pelvis in an upward and descending development.

Lap Dance

This is a great posture for a man to encounter his darling's body in the entirety of its magnificence. His hands will be allowed to meander around her body, and he can do what he needs. The lady will face away from him as she would have, had she been giving him a lap move. The man should sit down on a seat for playing out this represents, and his back should be kept straight. The lady will then sit on his lap and parity herself by setting her hands on his upper thighs or even his stomach. She will then need to lift herself gradually and place the backs of her calves and brings down herself onto his penis. Another variety of this would be that the lady should bring down herself onto his penis while confronting her darling. This will give him a serious decent perspective on her bosoms. He can choose to prod and play with them for whatever length of time that he satisfies.

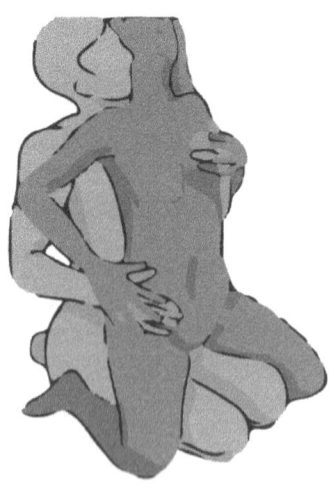

Pretzel

This is another representation that is satisfying to take a gander at and even simple to expect. This will cause the couple to feel incredibly attractive. For playing out this procedure, the couple should stop before one another. The man should move advances, and the lady will fold her arms over him. The lady will then lift herself and place her left leg by her darling's correct foot; her foot will confront downwards. The man will then need to put his left leg close to her correct foot. When taken a gander at a couple occupied with this posture, they look like a pretzel, an extremely provocative and mouth-watering pretzel.

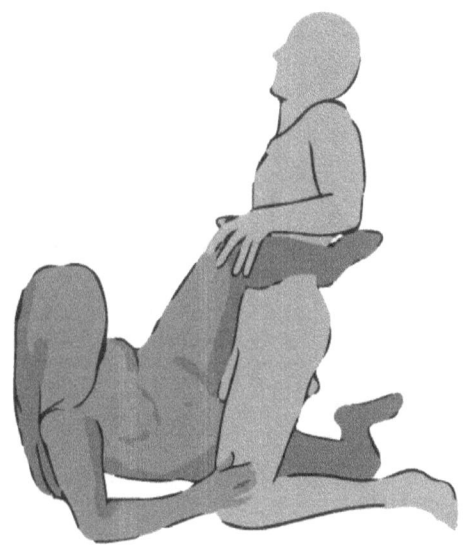

The Spread

This is an essential and amazingly hot position. This permits the lady to get incredible delight since it lets her stroke her sweetheart and permits him the entrance to joy her. For playing out this system, the lady should sit at the very edge of the couch or even the bed and spread her legs separated. The man will then need to remain in the middle of her legs and infiltrate her. She can draw nearer to him and kiss him while his hands have her full body entrance.

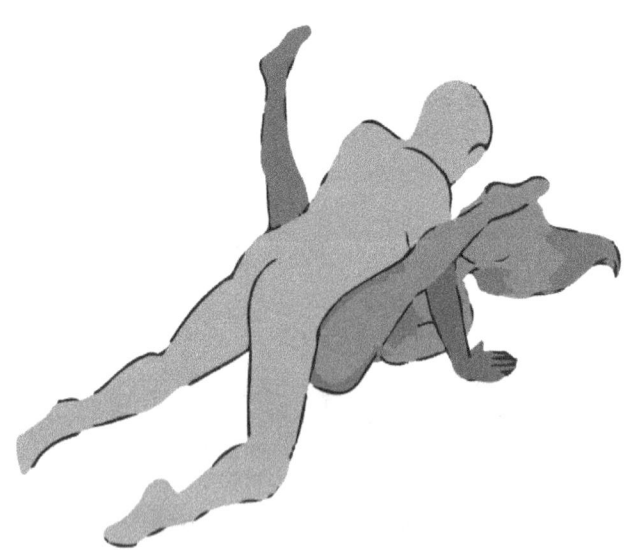

The Entwine

This posture looks intense and about difficult to copy, however, then it very well may be pleasurable if it's done appropriately. This posture is tastefully engaging. For playing out this strategy, the couple should sit near one another and face each other. The man should put his legs on either side of his partner. The lady will then need to lift both of her legs and place them on either side of her sweetheart's sides, under his arms. The man's upper arms will secure the lady's legs, and the lady will then need to lift her upper arms and place them over his elbows. The man will then lift his legs and place them over her hands. This does sound very messy, isn't that right? All the exertion that goes into it will merit your time and energy.

The G-force

This is maybe one of the most blazing tantric sex presents there is. This is the piece de opposition of all sex presents. The man has full oversight over his darling right now. Both the people included will get extraordinary delight from this posture. For playing out this position, the lady should rest on her back on the bed, and the man must bow by her legs. He will then gradually lift her middle off the bed so she's offsetting herself with her head and her shoulders put on the bed. The man can either extend her legs at a 90-degree edge or infiltrate her, or he can likewise pull them separated and place her feet just beneath his chest and enter her.

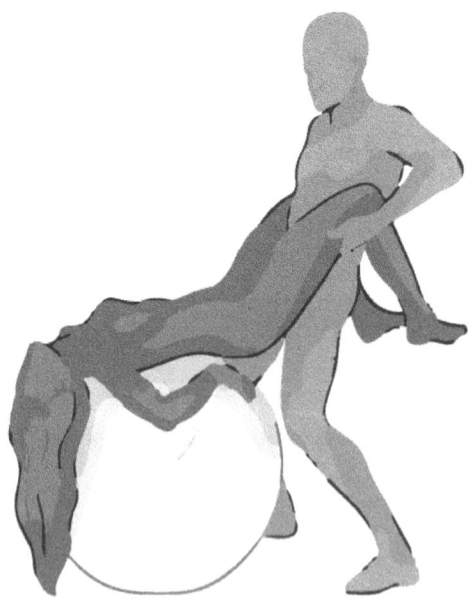

The Waterfall

Right now, a lady should put her hand on her sweetheart's penis and afterward let her fingertips brush his scrotum gradually and tenderly. It is a smart thought to use some ointment for making it progressively pleasurable. Her hands should be set on either side of his gonads, and afterward, she should gradually slide her hands up till they arrive at the touchy tip of his penis. When this is done, the lady should give the man some time to chill off, and he will then need to respond to the administration he got. The man needs to cup his sweetheart's vagina and touch all her delicate spots. He should slide his hands over her clitoris and her vaginal external lips.

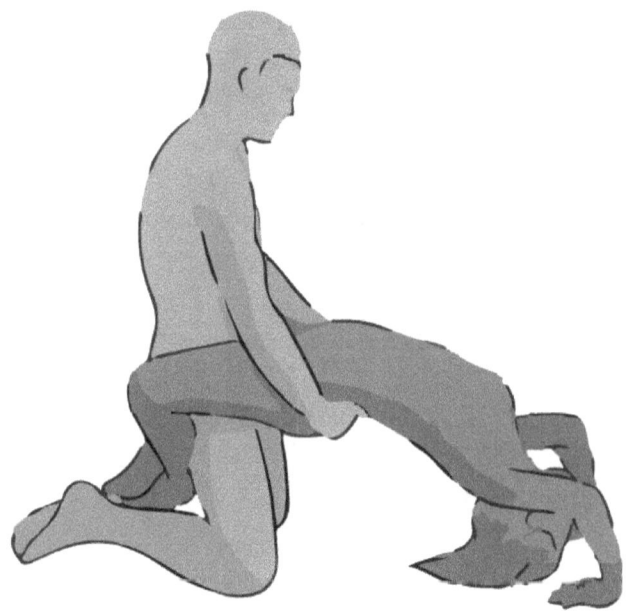

The Snake

For this, the lady should gradually extend the pole of her sweetheart's penis with one of her hands and let the other hand follow little circles directly under the leader of the pole. This is like giving slow and delicate handwork.

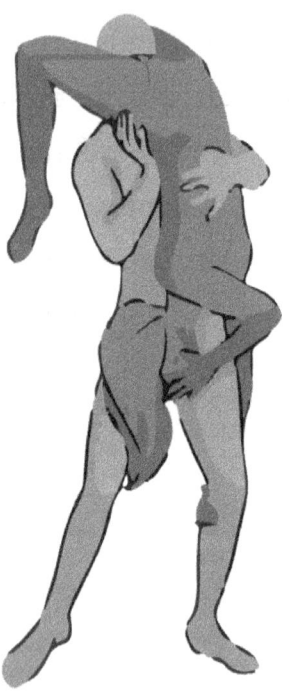

CHAPTER 11:

Multiple Orgasm

The orgasm has long been viewed as the peak of sexual excitement. It's a very powerful feeling of pleasure, which involves releasing accumulated erotic tension. While everybody's goal with sex is an orgasm, there isn't a lot known about it. During the last few centuries, theories about the orgasm have changed. For example, experts have only recently started talking about female orgasm. Many doctors in the 1970s claimed that it was perfectly normal for a woman not to experience an orgasm.

Orgasms can be defined in several ways with different criteria. Medical professionals talk about physiological changes that happen within the body. Mental health professionals and psychologists talk about cognitive and emotional changes. There is not a single, overarching definition of the orgasm.

Sex researchers have tried to define orgasms in models of sexual response. While the process for orgasm can differ between people, several basic physiological changes often occur in most incidences.

Master and Johnson's Four-Phase Model includes:

- Excitement
- Plateau
- Orgasm
- Resolution

Kaplan came up with his model, but he differs from most sexual response models because it includes desire. The majority of models don't include non-genital changes. It's important to understand, though, that not every sexual act is preceded by desire. Kaplan's three-stage model is:

- Desire
- Excitement
- Orgasm

Benefits of Orgasms

A 1997 cohort suggested that men's mortality risk was lowered when they experienced a high number of orgasms than in men who had fewer orgasms. There is also some research that suggests ejaculation can help to reduce the risk of prostate cancer. Researchers found that a man's prostate cancer risk was 20% lower in those who ejaculated at least 21 times a month than those who ejaculated only four to seven times a month.

There are a lot of hormones that are released during orgasm, which includes DHEA and oxytocin. Some studies suggest these hormones may help protect against heart disease and certain cancers. Oxytocin, as well as other endorphins that are released during the female and male orgasm, are also relaxants.

Types of Orgasm

Not surprisingly, since experts haven't reached a consensus regarding a definition of an orgasm, there are many different types of orgasms. Sigmund Freud stated that female orgasms as clitoral in immature and young, and vaginal in women with a healthy sexual response. In contrast to this, Betty Dodson has said that at least nine different orgasms are biased towards genital stimulation. We'll go over a few of those types.

- Tension orgasms – This is a common type of orgasm. It is created through direct stimulation, often when the muscles and body are tense.

- Relaxation orgasms – This orgasm comes from deep relaxation through sexual stimulation.

- Pressure orgasms – This orgasm comes from indirect stimulation of applied pressure. This is a type of self-stimulation that is common in young people.

- Multiple orgasms – These are a series of orgasms that happen over a short period.

- Blended or combination orgasms – These are a variety of orgasmic experiences that blend together.

There are a few orgasms that both Dodson and Freud discounted, but others believe they are real. For example:

- G-spot orgasms – This is an orgasm that is caused by the stimulation of an erotic zone in the vagina through penetrative intercourse, which feels very different from orgasms caused by other forms of stimulation.

- Fantasy orgasm – These are orgasms that result from mental stimulation.

The Female Orgasm

Men and women go through similar yet different physiological processes when experiencing an orgasm. Here we will talk about the process of the female orgasm following the Masters and Johnson four-phase model.

1. **Excitement**

    When a woman is psychologically or physically stimulated, the blood vessels in her genitals will dilate. This increased blood flow will make the vulva swell, and fluid will pass through the vaginal walls.

This makes the vulva wet and swollen. Internally, the vagina expands at the top. Breathing and heart rate will quicken, and her blood pressure will rise. The blood vessel dilation can cause a woman to look flushed, especially on the chest and neck.

2. **Plateau**

As the blood flows to the lower vagina area, it will reach a limit and turn firm. Breasts can also increase in size by 25% and increase the blood to the areola, making the nipples look less erect. The clitoris will then pull back against the pubic bone, making it look like it has disappeared.

3. **Orgasm**

The genital muscles will experience rhythmic contractions that are about 0.8 seconds apart. For women, their orgasms last longer at about 13 to 51 seconds. Since women don't have a recovery period, they can continue to experience orgasms if stimulated again.

4. **Resolution**

The body will slowly return to its previous state, reducing breathing, pulse rate, and swelling.

The Male Orgasm

1. **Excitement**

   When a man experiences psychological or physical stimulation, he gets an erection. Blood flow increased in the corpora, which is the tissue that runs throughout the penis, which causes the penis to grow and become hard. The testicles will draw up as the scrotum tightens.

2. **Plateau**

   With the increased blood flow, the testicles and glans will increase in size. The buttock and thigh muscles will tense, the pulse quickens, blood pressure rises, and breathing increases.

3. **Orgasm**

   Semen, a mixture of 95% fluid and 5% sperm, is forced through the urethra by contractions in the pelvic floor, vas deferens, seminal vesicles, and prostate glands. These contractions also cause the semen to be forced out of the penis, causing ejaculation. Orgasm for a man tends to last for ten to 30 seconds.

4. **Resolution**

The man is now in the recovery phase, where he can't have any more orgasms. This is what is called a refractory period, and how long it lasts varied between men. It could be a few minutes to a few days and tends to become longer the older the man becomes. At this point, the testicles and penis return to their original size. Their pulse and breathing will be fast.

Multiple Orgasms

People find the idea of multiple orgasms intriguing and for a good reason. It is perfectly normal to want to experience one right after the other and simply tapping out after the first. Here, we will discuss why the female body is designed to experience multiple orgasms, and strategies to make them more likely to happen.

Having multiple orgasms doesn't necessarily mean that you have another orgasm right after your first one without a moment's rest, but you can do that. Multiple orgasms simply mean that you have several orgasms during a single sexual encounter.

To experience multiple orgasms, will require some experimentation on your part. After you have your first, you will need to figure out what can make it happen again. If you find that your clitoris is so sensitive that you can't touch it, use the rest of your body. Try out different forms of stimulation. This could be playing with your breasts or getting your partner to kiss everything except the clitoris. The main point is to continue the arousal in whatever way works for you. Continue this for however long you want. You can always check back in with the clitoris to see if some of the sensitivity has gone away.

That being said, sometimes stimulating the sensitive clitoris could be the ticket. Some women say continuing to run the clitoris gives them the chance to embrace what seems like unbearable overstimulation, which can result in more orgasms. It all depends on what you can handle. If you like oversensitivity, then do it. If it hurts or can't see it creating a pleasurable feeling, don't continue touching it just to try and have more orgasms.

You can also use Kegal exercises to help extend your orgasms. As you reach your first orgasm, push your hand over your vulva and pulse it between orgasm contractions as you squeeze your thighs. Doing this can intensify and increase the orgasmic contraction and bring you into another orgasm.

You also need to make sure that you breathe during the entire experience. There are some people who will unconsciously hold their breath as the orgasm builds, but concentrating can help. When you reach or orgasm, breath purposefully, slowly, and deeply while contracting your pelvic floor muscles. This breathwork can lead to multiples for some people.

These tips are a great place to start but don't get upset if they don't work the first time. It takes practice and learning your body.

CHAPTER 12:

Tips to Improve Tantric Sex

More often than not, when an orgasm is achieved, it will be by one party or the other. It is fairly rare for both people to achieve orgasm at the same time. There may have been occurrences where this has happened for you and your partner. Still, it was likely not on purpose, and repeating it, if you tried, was probably quite difficult.

We will provide you with information on how you and your partner can work together so that you can orgasm together. If you have never experienced a mutual orgasm with your lover, it is something for the record books. Many couples have heard about this but have never experienced it. By gaining some information, you will likely be able to climax together and share an experience unlike any other.

Having an orgasm at the same time as your partner will truly deepen your connection. You will likely be more in love with them than ever before when you can experience something like this. When our body's orgasm, they release hormones; if this occurs simultaneously, it will help both of you become more in tune with the other. It cannot only enhance your sex life but also your relationship.

You want to keep in mind that it takes women longer to reach orgasm than it does men. By implementing extra foreplay, you can make it easier for your lady. Clitoral stimulation is a great way to help her achieve orgasm more easily. One way to provide extra sensation to her clitoris is for her to cross her legs while you are in just about any position. It will slow things down, which will make him last longer, and it will also allow his pelvis and member to stimulate the clitoris.

A big part of reaching orgasm together is to slow everything down. Men tend to reach orgasm when they have deep penetration and arrhythmic style of stimulation. If you notice he is getting close, the best thing you can do is limit his penetration level and slow everything down to a turtle's pace. The female will likely want to be the one in control of this as when he is close to orgasm, he may not think about it. Communication is also going to play a role, make sure your partner is letting you know if they're getting close. This will allow you to decide if you are close enough to make it to or if you need to slow things down and make the process longer.

Eye contact during intercourse is also critical. This is especially true if you are trying to orgasm together. When we can look into each other's eyes, it is a very intimate thing. It also gives off a very good set of nonverbal cues that allows your partner to understand when you are getting close to the climax. The fact that eye contact can be difficult to maintain, but with practice, it becomes easier. Taking the time to get comfortable looking into each other's eyes for long periods can make it easier for the two of you to orgasm together.

Allowing the woman to be in control is also advantageous. Because her orgasm is going to take longer, allowing her to be in control will let her set the pace so that you guys have a chance of orgasming together. The best positions to do this would-be one like cowgirl or her straddling him on a chair. The motion that works the best for her will be achieved in these types of positions. Additionally, they allow for easy clitoral stimulation. As we know, double stimulation for a female makes achieving orgasm a much simpler thing.

If simultaneous orgasm is the goal, you should never be afraid to stop. Simply stopping it while intercourse is still happening can be nearly impossible when we are close to climax. If you notice your partner is getting close, but you still need more time simply stop the activity. Spend some time kissing, cuddling, and caressing each other. This can help to calm things down but still, keep your partner aroused. After things have settled down and orgasm is no longer ready to happen, you can continue having sex. This tactic can be implemented at any point during your lovemaking sessions.

Something that may take a little practice but can be super helpful is when men learn to do Kegel muscle exercises. Sure, this is a thing that most women are already doing to make sure that they have strong pelvic floor muscles and that they feel tight during penetration. Men have the same muscles on their pelvic floor. When these muscles are strengthened, they can help him last longer. If your man is about to reach orgasm, have him perform an extended Kegel muscle exercise and take a few deep breaths. More often than not, this will help the urge to climax subside. Additionally, the more he practices this technique, the better it will work.

Speaking of Kegel muscles, they can also be utilized by the female. If a woman performs Kegel muscle tightening during intercourse, it can help her reach climax faster. It helps to build arousal because of the increased blood flow to the area that these exercises cause. The feeling of this can also be quite stimulating for the man. The bottom line is that everyone should be doing Kegel muscle exercises inside and outside the bedroom. They are a good variety of benefits to doing so.

The motions that you use during intercourse will also play a major role. Many men find that the in and out motion gets them and allows them to reach climax easily. So, by switching up the motion so that it is rocking or grinding rather than thrusting in and out, you can make him last a lot longer, giving the female more time for her orgasm to build up. Rocking motions are fantastic as they also allow for clitoral stimulation regardless of the position you may be in. So, even if your hands aren't free, get to rocking and realize how quickly you can achieve orgasm together.

Don't be afraid to provide yourself with extra stimulation if you need to achieve orgasm. This goes for the man or the woman. Clitoral stimulation is always going to help a woman achieve orgasm more quickly but paying attention to other erogenous zones of the body can also be beneficial. Maybe your man has an extremely sensitive spot on his shoulder, or he is into anal stimulation by paying attention to these areas you can get your partner going. Conversations and paying attention to each other can help you both understand the best ways to ensure that simultaneous orgasms can happen from time to time.

Another great thing to keep in mind if you are trying to orgasm together is that adding pressure to the base of a man's penis can help stop his orgasm in its tracks. Whether his female counterpart does it or he does it himself, trying to stop an orgasm can be made a bit easier by using this tactic. When you are truly in the moment, it can be a bit hard to remember, but it'll be worth the time to implement this.

You must understand that if you are going to have a simultaneous orgasm with your partner, it will not be during a one-night stand. You need to know the person and be able to read their cues to make it happen. When you understand their physical responses and how their body reacts before orgasm, it provides you with the information you need to stop or keep going. Mutual orgasms are a thing of trial and error. It is likely you will need to keep at it to make it happen and tweak things so that each time you get closer to it happening.

There is no rush in making this type of thing happen. It just takes practice and communication. Discussing your sex session after it happens and figuring out what you can do to prolong the session to the point of you climaxing together is advantageous. Don't get stressed out if you can't make it happen right away, instead enjoy the time you get to spend with your partner trying.

Another trick that can help you achieve a simultaneous orgasm is almost as good as eye contact. We're talking about synchronizing your breathing. Synchronizing your breath with another person does take a bit of time. The best way to do it is in a position where the female's back is against the male's chest. This will allow her to feel him breathe and make her breathing pattern the same. It is amazing how intimate it is when you start to breathe in the same rhythm as your partner. By maintaining this matched breath achieving mutual orgasm is significantly easier.

Sometimes it's hard for people to find the words they want while in the throes of passion. You can come up with a fun code for you and your partner so that there is a mutual understanding of how close to climax each of you is. You can do this with simple things like squeezing each other's hands or how you touch each other can change. It can be quite fun coming up with the system, so the other one knows if you are only 50% of the way there or if you are right around the corner from achieving orgasm.

All in all, you need to remember that intercourse with your partner is supposed to be fun. It should not be a stressful situation. Sure, achieving mutual orgasm is something that everyone wants to experience, but it does take some time and practice. Stay calm and know eventually you guys will be able to get there together.

Once you have been able to climax together, it is likely that you are going to want to do it again. Trying the same tactics may be the best avenue to ensure that you can repeat the process. However, spicing things up and doing things differently each time can also be advantageous. It keeps both parties on their toes and can make having sex more fun in the long run.

Conclusion

Tantric sex positions' is an excellent short fictional story that will allow you to see the tantric sex practice from various perspectives. The tantric sex practice does not need any fabrication to make it appear valid. It is reasonable, as it is stated. It can show you how to feel the energy in the body before any actual sexy action happens.

The Tantric sex practice is about developing the interconnectedness of the universe. It creates a robust and energetic connection.

Tantric sex helps in learning how to feel the energy in the body before it acts. This is part of intelligent sexual development.

Tantric sex practice does not require any physical intercourse action. All Tantric sex practices are based on the inner story and not on the action happening externally. Tantric sex teaches people about the fullness of the sexual pleasure experienced by connecting the sexual organs in a certain way.

The Tantric sex practice in itself does not need an orgasm to happen as sometimes people think. This is not a cock and ball or pussy and cock kind of act. This does not require penetration. Sexual organs are not present in Tantric sex practices, but they are utilized.

An orgasm can be experienced by practicing Tantric sex practice if practicing in different positions and comfortable and relaxed enough.

When practicing Tantric sex in conjunction with pure sexual practices, an orgasm can be experienced.

Some people think that Tantric Sex is an Ejaculation kind of sex, but this is not true as the orgasms taken after Tantric sex practice are not meant for cock and balls ejaculation. Still, they are meant for experiencing and understanding the body.

Some involuntary actions often accompany the non-ejaculatory orgasms that occur with the Tantric sex practice. This might happen only once in a lifetime, during the Tantric sex practice.

Tantric sex can be practiced with a partner and without a partner. It is based on internal energies and not on the physical act happening externally.

The tantric process is devoted to discovering energy at its highest level through the various practices of yoga, meditation, and other disciplines. The methods are then used to develop the strength and help move it from the lower chakras to the highest chakra, the crown chakra, in the head's back.

Practicing tantric sex is also an exercise in creating a beautiful energy flow. It is an art form. We are living, breathing, organic sculptures... dynamic, vital, sensuous. Sex in itself is an art form. The following scenarios are meant to be simply suggestions — ways to bring tantric sex into your intimate life. They do not prescribe any specific actions or techniques but simply provide some starting points. Just follow the natural direction of your instincts. You are the artist, the breath, the beauty.

As you practice and learn the simplicity of this approach, you may be astounded by how it helps you and your partner experience a level of intimacy that you never thought was possible. And I am not just talking about the emotional and spiritual side of sex. I am talking about all the aspects of sexual pleasure.

You will notice that tantric sex doesn't necessarily require penetration, or orgasm, or ejaculation. Ejaculation can often hinder the fullness of sexual experience. If you are engaged in tantric sex, then you can develop many different tantric sex practices without the need for "coming."

Yet you can easily add those practices as you progress. And if they feel right, simply intensify them. How you experience sex depends on several factors that can change over time. How's your health? How easily can you relax? How much sexual experience do you have? How available is your partner? How much time do you have?

But whatever those variables, tantric sex can be a most profound and intimate experience, one that requires nothing more than you and your partner, your bodies, your breath, your consciousness, and each other.

www.ingramcontent.com/pod-product-compliance
Lightning Source LLC
Chambersburg PA
CBHW070920080526
44589CB00013B/1380